THE BLAME GAME

THE BLAME GAME

SHIFTING FROM PROBLEMS TO SOLUTIONS

Simple and easy to understand insights into
the subconscious mind of self-limiting patterns.
Go from surviving to thriving with some quick shifts
in perception of yourself and the world around you.

KATHLEEN PLEASANTS

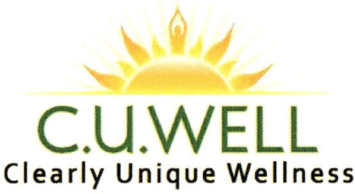

Copyright © Kathleen Pleasants, 2019

All Rights Reserved

No part of this book may be reproduced in any form, by photocopying or by any electronic or mechanical means, Including information storage or retrieval systems, without permission in writing from both the copyright owner and the publisher of this book.

Cover and Design by Paula A. Faccio

First Published 2019 by Clearly Unique Wellness

TABLE OF CONTENTS

Dedication vi

Acknowledgments vii

Foreword viii

Introduction ix

CHAPTER ONE: The Blame Game 13

CHAPTER TWO: Law of Attraction................................... 19

CHAPTER THREE: Judgment... 21

CHAPTER FOUR: From Anger to Hope 23

CHAPTER FIVE: Never Say Never 29

CHAPTER SIX: Look Around You, What Do You See?.... 31

CHAPTER SEVEN: A Shift in Perspective......................... 35

Conclusion xxxix

About the Author xli

DEDICATION

I dedicate this book
to all who appreciate
simple reminders that life is good
and to those who want to live
the best life they can!

ACKNOWLEDGMENTS

Paula A. Faccio - Lead Editor & Designer

Damon Kinnaman - Graphic Designer

Derrick Acosta - For his critiquing and helpful suggestions

FOREWORD

Mindfulness. This simple practice seems to be among the most difficult feats of mankind. To be "in the moment" and be aware of our own feelings and what these feelings do in us. This is due to fear; fear of what our strong emotions will reveal about us. Do we dare explore our most inward thoughts and allow ourselves to feel the emotions? The prospect of self-reflection may seem overwhelming but when the courage to explore these depths is taken, we then find true freedom and Joy ready to embrace us.

Gratefulness. This has the power to revolutionize any circumstance. It can take a person from the depths of depression to the heights of healing in a split moment and a slight shift in thought can melt away despair. In my psychotherapy practice, I have continually seen this phenomenon which allows a suffering soul to find peace. The marriage of mindfulness and courage bring this gratefulness which is the remedy to bio-psycho-social-spiritual brokenness.

Kathleen Pleasants in The Blame Game exposes the barriers to finding more peace and living a life of unlimited potential and fulfillment. It sheds light on the understanding that we hold more power than we believe and have the control to bring our thoughts captive through practical steps which can free our spirits and allow us to live in freedom.

~ Kelly Kaitson, LCSW.

INTRODUCTION

There are some people that will never trust enough to allow themselves to live more freely; to live and let live. It seems like such a simple task. Allow your true freedom to re-enter a little bit at a time and you'll make great progress towards living the fullest life available to you.

Pay attention to your thoughts, good or not good. Lead any negative thought in a positive direction as soon as you are aware of it.

Start by changing your thought process in small ways. Once you get used to this, you'll find it is easier to redirect your thoughts in a positive direction. The goal is to see things differently. Let those positive thoughts build as long as you possibly can. This exercise has the force to move mountains and can be used to create the world you want. In time you can shift the bigger non-serving thoughts more quickly.

One step at a time gets you there.

No matter what anyone tells you, always try what feels right to you and see how that works out. That is all you are asked to do in this lifetime.

Pause, and wait until you feel an inspiration from within. Move from moment to moment into what feels best and learn to expect the best around every corner.

THE BLAME GAME

Breathe deeply, feel Joyful and bask in this feeling daily.

What I am writing is not new. My perspective may be a bit unique, but what you are about to read has been said and practiced in many ways before.

You can find many books on the topic of Law of Attraction that will bring more light to what flows closely to your heart.

I am only sharing my perspective from my own experience and practice with this universal law of our existence. I am simply intending to save my breath in trying to explain to others why they may continually re-create the same types of situations over and over again into their lives. I give examples of how that may happen and how they can shift their thoughts; which will change their experiences once-and-for-all for the better.

I don't just talk about these setups to shutting down much of one's potential, but I list ways to move into finding more peace and fulfillment through gentle practices that can become one's Daily Habits.

Within these pages you will find ways to clean out the corners of your life and the under-carpet sweepings that create bumps and stumbles that get in the way. You now have the chance to reach your goals at your own pace without the opinion of others contributing to detours along the way.

I believe wholeheartedly that life is meant to be good, fun and rich. Each day gives us huge opportunities for growth and re-creation, whether that is through working with others or time alone.

SHIFTING FROM PROBLEMS TO SOLUTIONS

Christ said, "No man can enter heaven unless he is like a child." If you lose the wonder of really noticing all the good that surrounds you, then you lose the sight of Heaven on Earth. Being in a physical body is the ultimate gift and trying to get out of it or ignoring it will show you what Hell is truly like. Heaven and Hell exists here on Earth and you are given the freedom to choose one or the other daily, even moment by moment.

Read on and find reminders of how you can find your true freedom and wonderment that has never left you and is ready to explore new paths of discovery no matter your age or beliefs.

CHAPTER ONE

THE BLAME GAME

> "Brad, Brad bo-bad, banana fanna fo-fad,
> fee-fi mo-mad, Br-a-a-d."
> (From the song, The Name Game)

Is Brad responsible for the way you feel? Barbara? Terry? Charlie? How about the neighbor? The dog? The car? If all these things can be responsible for your unhappiness, then what in the world do you have control over?

If you are always making it someone else's fault that things aren't going well for you, then you are playing *The Blame Game*. Do you realize that no one ever wins at this game? You don't feel better for long before the next thing to blame comes along. In these cases, the faces and places may change but the pattern is always the same – Blame.

If you want to feel better, stop playing the blame game. Listen to what you are saying and pay attention to how you are feeling when

CHAPTER ONE

something irritating happens and pulls all of your attention to it. Are you quick to attach a name and leave yourself out of it? If you feel upset with someone or something, you are fully in the game.

In the case of the blame game, once you have stopped playing, you will find that you have the energy to approach any problem in a new way.

We miss so many opportunities to make changes and to live in harmony with others because we don't want to take the time to clean up our thoughts and to look for another way in the moment, and so we proceed purely out of habit.

I see a lot of verbal and physical abuse from people who are constantly badgering others over what they did or didn't do. In the meantime, nothing improves and there is a lot of energy-slinging that could have been used to accomplish something better. Either let it go or make the change yourself.

Don't ever expect others to read your mind or behave like you. Realize that at times, when you make a request, you are asking or demanding another to do something you don't want to do; yet you expect others to jump for you. That's a very contradictory energy aimed at another.

Check out the following list for how the Blame Game is played. If you use one or all of these excuses, (on the left side), you will want to play *The Change Game,* (on the right side), to get out of Blame all together:

THE BLAME GAME

The Blame Game	**The Change Game**
He did/ She did...	He did/ She did, So What?
It's not my fault...	I attract all that comes to me in my life.
They should have known better...	It is not for me to judge what others choose.
I can't do this without their help...	I could find others that are willing to help; it doesn't always have to be the ones that are close to me.
I have tried and tried to tell them...	I can only control my own life.
If things were different... How can I get it through to them?	Things can be different, I'm not responsible for others.
They always find a way to get out of this...	I can find another way to get this done.
Will they ever change?	I can only change myself.
It figures, they get hurt just when I need them...	I choose to focus on what's working.
No one is ever there for me.	What I feel is what I feel; I can stop blaming others for how I feel.
This always happens.	I can let myself off the hook. Resolve is around the corner.
I wish I were different.	I am fine with where and who I am.
If I were in a different house, had a different job, had more money, friends, time...	I can find a way to feel better about where I am.
If they would just listen.	If I step away, I can find a different solution.
If I don't tell them, how will they ever know?	That's just none of my business!

CHAPTER ONE

Feel the energy that is given off by blame and imagine what else you would do if you could harness that and use it for something more productive and rewarding.

You have the tools you need to get out of a bad space. You know you must take your focus off of whatever you are blaming and focus on any good that you can find in the situation or, if you can't do that, just think of something that makes you feel better for now; Anything! Once again, you must concentrate on something better. What's best to remember is that, the tools stay the same, it is only the situations that change. However, if you don't understand and identify the situations that cause you to feel badly, then you will get caught in an endless loop of feeling frustrated and wondering why.

Half of being able to change is having the ability to know what you need to change.

> Repeating a pattern of blame makes me think of the quote by Narcotics Anonymous, 1981...
>
> "The very definition of insanity is to keep doing the same thing over and over again, expecting different results."

Once you are in a better space, you will have the energy to try another way and you may even realize a completely different solution that resolves the whole issue.

Even though *The Blame Game* is a common pastime for many, it doesn't feel good and it doesn't create a space for new views and answers. Once you have stopped playing, you will find that you have the ability to take the spin off of recurring issues with these new self-empowerment tools.

~ GIVE IT A TRY ~

The Change Game will bring you so many rewards and so much gratitude as well as happy times. It is never too late to bring the *no blame* harmony into your family dynamics and into your life.

Now Brad can be let off the hook.

Make statements of
what you want
and make it a point to believe them.

CHAPTER TWO

LAW OF ATTRACTION

Try to understand that you have attracted many situations into your life that you are now trying to fight away or run away from, but they have no choice but to follow your magnet that has drawn them there.

Wherever you go, you take yourself with you. The same situations can pop up easily and the same dramas will creep in no matter how far you run. In the law of attraction, there is nowhere to run or hide and no one to get away from, but only the need to change your inner ways. If you don't like what's around you, a bit of rearranging may do the trick for a while, but it won't go away unless you rearrange your thoughts from the inside and take a hold of being a *conscious creator.* With making how you feel a priority; there is always an opportunity for a better way.

It's amazing how you can take any situation and find the good in it, around it, behind it and/or through it. You can take a past experience and do the same with it. It's even easier to imagine a future one with

CHAPTER TWO

a better ending. Sometimes you have to start in the future, to find a way to feel better, before you can find the rewards that are around you now.

Try seeing life as an eye spy game; you are looking at a big picture with a huge amount of details and you only need to find a few strategically placed objects to win. Consider looking for more of the good in the world as hidden objects that are always there just waiting to be found so that you can feel better in just being able to see them. As with any other game, you will get better at this over time.

CHAPTER THREE

JUDGMENT

Judgment is a type of complaining and blame. You are still saying something is wrong with this picture. In the Law of Attraction, your reality only presents reflections of your own thoughts. Mostly you are trying to project these irritants you don't like onto others to feel better. You are actually trying to fight against and are ignoring your own self. You have heard, *it takes one to know one,* right? These are the types of people and situations you are attracting in; a perfect match to where you are mentally and physically.

Make peace with other's choices and watch what starts showing up around you. You'll be making peace with your own self. You will be very pleased indeed.

Consider others that seem to irritate you as gifts and an opportunity to check-in with yourself and what you need to release internally.

When you see something that throws you into judgment, say, "Okay, so I am judging this situation but… I can turn it around to a better topic." Don't even blame yourself for the thoughts. Make peace with

CHAPTER THREE

the moment and feel the relief. It will get faster and easier with practice. Your judgments will lessen and a lot more fun will take its place. :)

In my experience, if you get intolerant or critical of situations or others, you may wind up with a rash or a physical irritation at some point.

Skin irritations and allergies are a sign of being intolerant of what's going on around you and/or your surroundings. Bach Flower Essences: Impatiens, Beech, Holly and other emotional remedies can help raise the issues to your awareness and assist you into relaxing more easily into your world.

CHAPTER FOUR

FROM ANGER TO HOPE

Anger is an important emotion; it can be freeing. It is the first step out of the feeling of powerlessness and a relief from suppression and depression.

Without anger rising to bring back the fire into your life, you may stay in a limited state. You may remain in a semi-functional, survival mode.

Think about how anger and frustration move you from within. It is a way to find new strengths if you allow yourself to feel it and then shift out of it into frustration which can lead to Hope. It can take minutes or days, but it is important not to make excuses and shut it down.

Shutting down can lead to a very uncomfortable cycle; Suppression and Depression to Anger - back to Suppression.

Some would rather use medication or just shut down than express themselves fully. People don't like being around angry people. When we get angry around others, we have to make a choice. When you feel

CHAPTER FOUR

the pressure that comes from holding back, use it as fuel. Feel the anger and burn through it.

Of course, it's better to express this away from others, but if you are in a situation where the anger is rising, it is best to let it out in some way that is harmless to others and not care what they think.

EXERCISES:

- Allow the anger to surface. Let yourself be mad. Don't tell yourself that a "good" person or a "loving" person wouldn't feel this anger, because that's not true. EVERYONE feels anger.
- Once you have accepted your anger, you need to understand that it was showing you where you need to shift your thoughts. "This too shall pass" is a good saying to work with, as these things always do.
- Call your power back through pulling from empowering experiences; times where things were going well. Enter into thoughts of what could go well and times where things were better.
- Take some time to write down what is good in your life. Write down what works for you; what makes you happy.

When you are stressed, you are making wishes for change. Make a list of what you want in your life and then shift your thoughts to seeing that happen, instead, in your mind's eye. That's where you want your thoughts to be as often as possible.

FROM ANGER TO HOPE

The high amount of depression and obedience we see around us stems from people caring about what others think and believing in obligations they have to their families and society. None of these should be a reason to shut down. Life that is worthy of living has passion and freedom of expression. Those who don't like it will fall away and those who admire your desire to live fully will enter into your life.

If there is a concern that you will become a rude and uncaring person by expressing what you feel when you feel it, then you need to focus on the following point: The purpose of anger and frustration is to move you towards hope. When you find relief in expressing your anger, rather than suppressing it, you'll start aiming towards harmony and better feelings in a very short amount of time.

I ask you, when you are feeling good, do you want to harm anyone, say hurtful things or bring others down? Not likely. You feel good and all's right with the world. That is the goal, to get to the emotional freedom of self-expression and to lift a burden you thought was important. To let go of what others think and set yourself free. In that space you do not feel anger, just happy and grateful.

When you are able to understand that anger is a telling sign of holding yourself back, you will find yourself less angry and falling into suppression less often. The feeling won't last as long, and you'll know how to move through it. Anger is not necessary when you feel you can make choices that are right for you.

CHAPTER FOUR

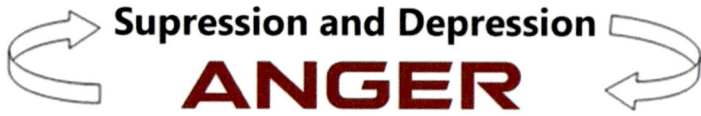

Supression and Depression ANGER

The 'Suppression and Depression to Anger – back to Suppression.' Cycle.

After you've owned your anger and have given yourself the right to feel it, now is the time to let it go and move onto something that makes you feel better. I know you've read that repeatedly throughout this book, but anger is a different emotion than others - which is why I chose to specifically address it.

- Feel your anger, let it move through you. Express your rage in whatever way you can without harm to yourself or others.
- Own the right to be angry!
- Move away from your anger into something that makes you feel better by finding an element that is positive in the situation or choose an entirely different thought that will help to lead you into a better perspective.

Use the pressure of holding back to power a rocket towards hope by using anger's fire to set a new course.

Anger is the rocket that promises to shoot you up into Hope. Take the ride, even though it may be rough at first, and try to appreciate this process to greater achievements.

For many, brief Anger is the ticket to relief and peace.

Let's appreciate and Respect its message.

FROM ANGER TO HOPE

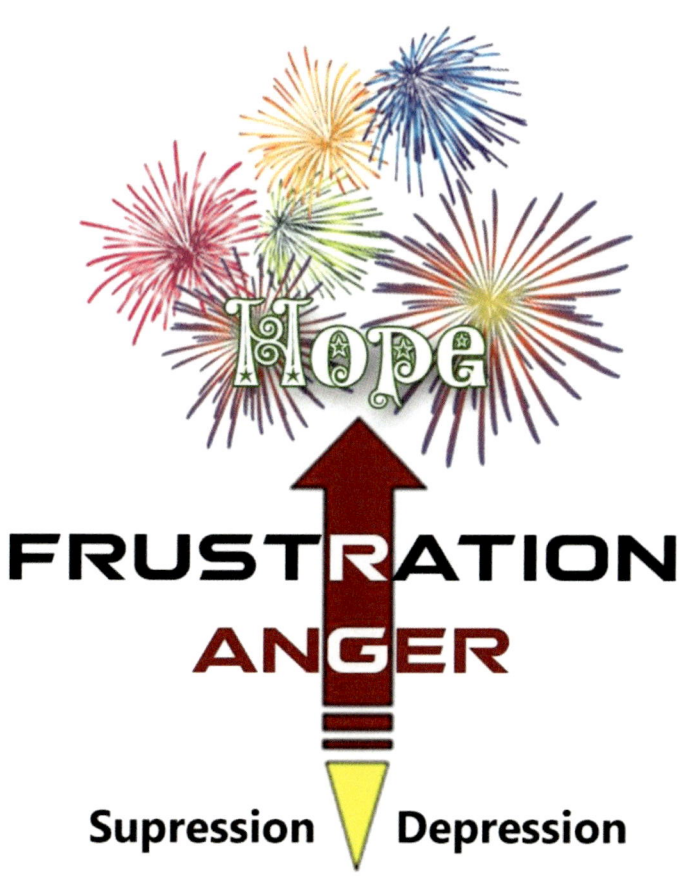

The outer limits of the Universe
and the inner limits within us
are all the same space.
You are limitless.

CHAPTER FIVE

NEVER SAY NEVER

Here's another view of how the Law of attraction works. Have you ever said *never* to something only to find that you actually wind up getting more of that? I used to say never to quite a few things. Without even knowing about the Law of Attraction, I would wind up inevitably attracting those types of situations into my life. I thought at the time that it was to help me to become more humble, but now I know it is the simple law of *what you focus on you get.* Just be careful what you say *never* to, especially if you repeat it and say it with emphasis.

Focus means focus no matter if it feels good or not good at all.

Spending time with a thought gives power to it whether wanted or not. You *never* know what better experiences await you in recognizing and shifting this pattern. All you have to do is resist judging others for what they do and focus on things that make you smile.

Daily Statement:

"On this day I choose to look for the good in my surroundings, in those that I meet and in what I am doing."

CHAPTER SIX

LOOK AROUND YOU, WHAT DO YOU SEE?

Your environment reflects where you are internally; your car, your home and the company you keep. Everything is an outward expression of your inner world (your thoughts and beliefs). Take inventory and notice what you are drawing into your world.

How well do things run for you, what condition is your house in, what is your car like? Start thinking of everything that surrounds you as put there by you; as a reflection of what you have chosen to focus on. Realize that what you see around you usually comes about by a *lack* of attention to what you are really feeling and creating from the inside.

We allow our thoughts to drive a course and we act as a passenger throughout our travels. We believe that things just happen to us and we are clueless to our contributions to every passing moment.

For days the place where I was staying had a temperamental shower. It would just go bloody hot in an instant without any warning. Of course, I wanted to blame this on the plumbing of the building, but

CHAPTER SIX

since I was writing a book on your outer environment expressing your inner environment, with no exceptions, I had no choice but to turn that temperament back onto myself.

I first thought, "What is the opposite of temperamental?" I figured it had to be consistency. I certainly wasn't being consistent and was running hot and cold in my daily life at that point.

As I recognized this within myself, I was able to build a comfortable relationship with the inconstancy that was there. I learned how to adjust the finicky shower handle, which for some reason I just couldn't figure out in the days prior, and was back in control of how to balance my life. I know I am given many outward hints into my patterns and habits that, if given acknowledgment, will lead me to wanted clarity and change.

Take a look at your luck too. How is that for you? Watch what you say about it. Everything can change for the better; you have to tell a better story to create new habits:

- So, I have lost things in the past but today is a new day and I have a chance to be more conscious of how I handle things.
- I have lent items of mine out that have never returned. I can appreciate that I have replaced many things in my life and have also received from others. It all works out and I can draw in people that are more conscious with my stuff so that I can enjoy the things I like longer and let them go if and when I choose to.

LOOK AROUND YOU, WHAT DO YOU SEE?

- I create my own luck by the stories I tell whether out loud or to myself. I always have the opportunity to tell another story or choose another topic that's more pleasing.

When you tell a story
you give it power,
only tell stories
you want to give power to.

CHAPTER SEVEN

A SHIFT IN PERSPECTIVE

Day to day challenges are something we all deal with. I remember a tough night I had with my children! And if I didn't take full responsibility for my feelings and the effort to turn it all around, it would have stayed that way. Instead, after I took the time to turn it around, it became one of the best nights I've had with them.

I knew I had to take myself out of the picture for a bit so that I could feel less overwhelmed and recoup. I knew that I was responsible for contributing to a dysfunctional rift. I needed a time-out before the night continued on that path; I had to change myself in order to change the situation.

My plan was to go into my room with the door shut and start to write positive aspects until I felt better.

When I got into the room it was dark, I didn't want to turn on any lights or even sit up to write at that moment. I just laid there in the dark trying to find some relief and then start writing. It wasn't long

CHAPTER SEVEN

before my son barged into the room saying something negative about what happened, then left. Just a couple of minutes later, he did the same thing. In spite of this, I was going to make a change.

A few more minutes past and I started to feel better, so I sat up, turned on the light, grabbed my notebook and pen and started to write:

<u>This is a nice room</u>
<u>We have a nice house</u>
<u>It's a blessing to be with all 3 of my kids</u>
<u>I can have a quiet space in here</u>
<u>Everyone is safe</u>
<u>I'm glad I can feel better...</u>

In walks my son again with another comment, but this time he closes the door behind him. I'm feeling a bit better, but still have a little way to go.

I continue:

<u>We have food in the pantry</u>
<u>I have a good reliable car outside</u>
<u>It's a nice neighborhood</u>
<u>We live by the woods</u>
<u>I have good neighbors...</u>

I don't remember all that I wrote that night, but that's basically how it goes when I write positive aspects. I try to simply focus on what's working and anything good I can think of at the time until I feel better.

It really works.

A SHIFT IN PERSPECTIVE

Then it happened, I felt better, I felt well enough to go back out. It only took about 10 or 15 minutes and I was done. I had shifted my energy and took responsibility for changing my mood; ultimately to change the situation.

I came out and went to check on my son. He was still a bit cranky, but was more tolerant and I was able to spend some positive time with him.

I went up to see my older daughter and sat down with her for a while to watch a show; we had a good time watching it.

Then I went over to my younger daughter and told her to go to the top of the stairs. I went downstairs and grabbed a small beach ball and threw it up to her. We spent a good amount of time playing catch; it was a lot of fun.

I was able to have quality time with each child. It seemed to all balance out well with my time and I have really fond memories of that night.

It turned out to be one of the most special nights with my kids.

...from the worst night, to the best night! All because I took the time to retreat and write positive aspects to change my perspective and the situation at hand.

It's our job to live
the best life ever;
to have time to cherish
the beautiful days and
the unending wonders
this life has to offer.
Somebody's gotta do it!

CONCLUSION

Everything I do is ultimately for me. Everything I have ever studied was my way of getting to know myself better. All my relationships and teachers were and are my mirrors. The more I learn, the closer I get to a deeper relationship and understanding of myself; removing veils and exposing hidden gems. You must get to know yourself, like one whom you adore, to get to truly see and be there for others.

If you gave a whole day to someone else, and also possibly didn't eat, or drink, or even sleep, you still did that for yourself. You believed that they were worthier and you believed in sacrifice and perhaps there would be a reward that you wouldn't typically come across without that experience. You were right. These were beliefs, not truths, and you still chose them. Whether it brought you Joy or sorrow, you were the one with the consequences; only you. Whatever the other person experienced was their own consequence; good or not good. You only have your path; shared with many others. But for those others, it's experienced in their own way based on their own beliefs.

In turning around the Blame Game to the Change Game, you realize that others will come and go and that you only have so much time per day, week and year to set goals and achieve them. Take time to write a *Mission Statement for your Life*. Don't make another decision without referring to it and holding true to your highest intension for yourself; every time!

THE BLAME GAME

The Simplicity of it all:
Think, Focus, Manifest

As you believe, you receive

How to write your Life Mission Statement:
https://www.clearlyuniquewellness.com/life-mission-statement

ABOUT THE AUTHOR

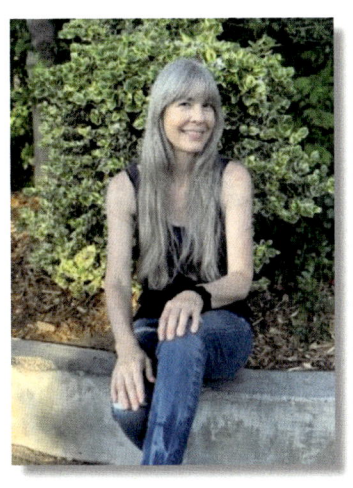

Kathleen Pleasants has been looking for spiritual, mental, emotional & physical answers since she was 10. "Why do people do what they do? What drives someone to say NO and not care what others think? How can some be so bold and others so shy? Why are some healthy and others not?" She never stopped asking these questions silently, but she did find her answers along the way and found peace in her own intentions. Kathleen learned, through trial and error, that we have always had a choice to look at things differently and choose another way if our way is not bringing us fulfillment. She formed Clearly Unique in 1991 where she practices Neuromuscular Therapy, Nutrition, Hypnotherapy, Grapho-therapy, Core Exercise and Coaching of Alternative Health Choices and Lifestyles with her clients. She became an Ordained Minister in 2001 through a two-year Interfaith Program in Pennsylvania.

Through the years she has traveled to many places to study with some of the top authorities in body, mind, emotional & physical modalities. She is the creator of the movie *Just My Type*, the Metabolic Typing Diet. She now travels nationally with her Unique Therapies &

THE BLAME GAME

Workshops and currently has her offices in San Diego, California.

You can learn more about Kathleen by visiting:
ClearlyUniqueWellness.com

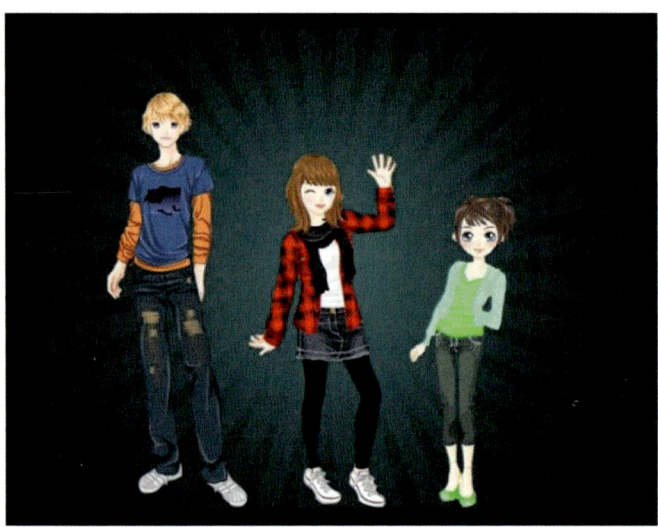

My Kids Make My Life RICH!

We each create our own world through our belief systems. Fortunately, beliefs can be changed and/or altered if we find ourselves in discomfort. We no longer have to get stuck in thoughts that make us feel guilty and depressed because we just can't live up to them. Go ahead, find freedom in making a new choice.

SHIFTING FROM PROBLEMS TO SOLUTIONS

Other books by Kathleen:

- EMOTIONS
- Our Daily Play
- Comfy Pants Chants
- JOY 20/20
- Awareness Activity Book
- Morning Journal Notebook
- Evening Journal Notebook
- Clearly Unique Journal Notebook
- Daily PLAY-by-PLAY Notebooks

You can find these books on Amazon

Made in the USA
Columbia, SC
02 February 2023